**FIRST U.S. EDITION**

**MOTIVATIONAL COACH & PUBLICIST:** Joy Cherry

ISBN-13: 978-1522813316

ISBN-10: 1522813314

# PREFACE

This book is an addendum to my book *Shape Shifting: The Alchemy of Losing Weight and Keeping It Off* which has as its target audience individuals who weigh 75 or more pounds over what is considered their normal weight (morbid obesity). While developing a marketing plan for the book I was reminded that morbid obesity frequently runs in families.

Often children of overweight adults whether, by genetics or socialization, become overweight at an early age and carry excess weight forward into adulthood. Teaching these children good eating habits, while educating their parents, could have a dramatic effect on obesity statistics in our society.

Therefore, this book has been set up in an easy-to-understand / easy-to-use format which can be fun for adults as well as children of all ages.

I invite you to get your colored pencils and crayons and become a kid again.

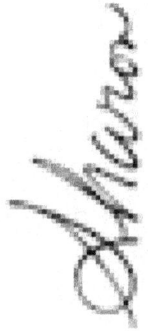

# Shape Shifter's Food Pyramid

COLOR ME RED (10%) - Foods to eat in moderation. They are good for you, but high in calories and point values. Examples include: Oils, nuts, grains (bread & pasta), avocados, sugars, dried fruits.

COLOR ME PINK (10%) - Cheese and dairy. Studies have determined that adult humans do not tolerate dairy well, as evidenced by growing reports of lactose intolerance. While dairy is a good source of calcium, there are non-dairy foods which are even better such as almond milk.

COLOR ME ORANGE (20%) - Lean proteins, including beans and vegetarian/vegan substitutes, eggs and cheese as a condiment (see above).

COLOR ME YELLOW (20%) - Starchy 1-2 point per serving vegetables. While quantities should be limited, they are a much healthier alternative than most breads and pastas when eaten with a meal.

COLOR ME GREEN (40%) - All fruit and 0-point vegetables which can be consumed in unlimited quantities.

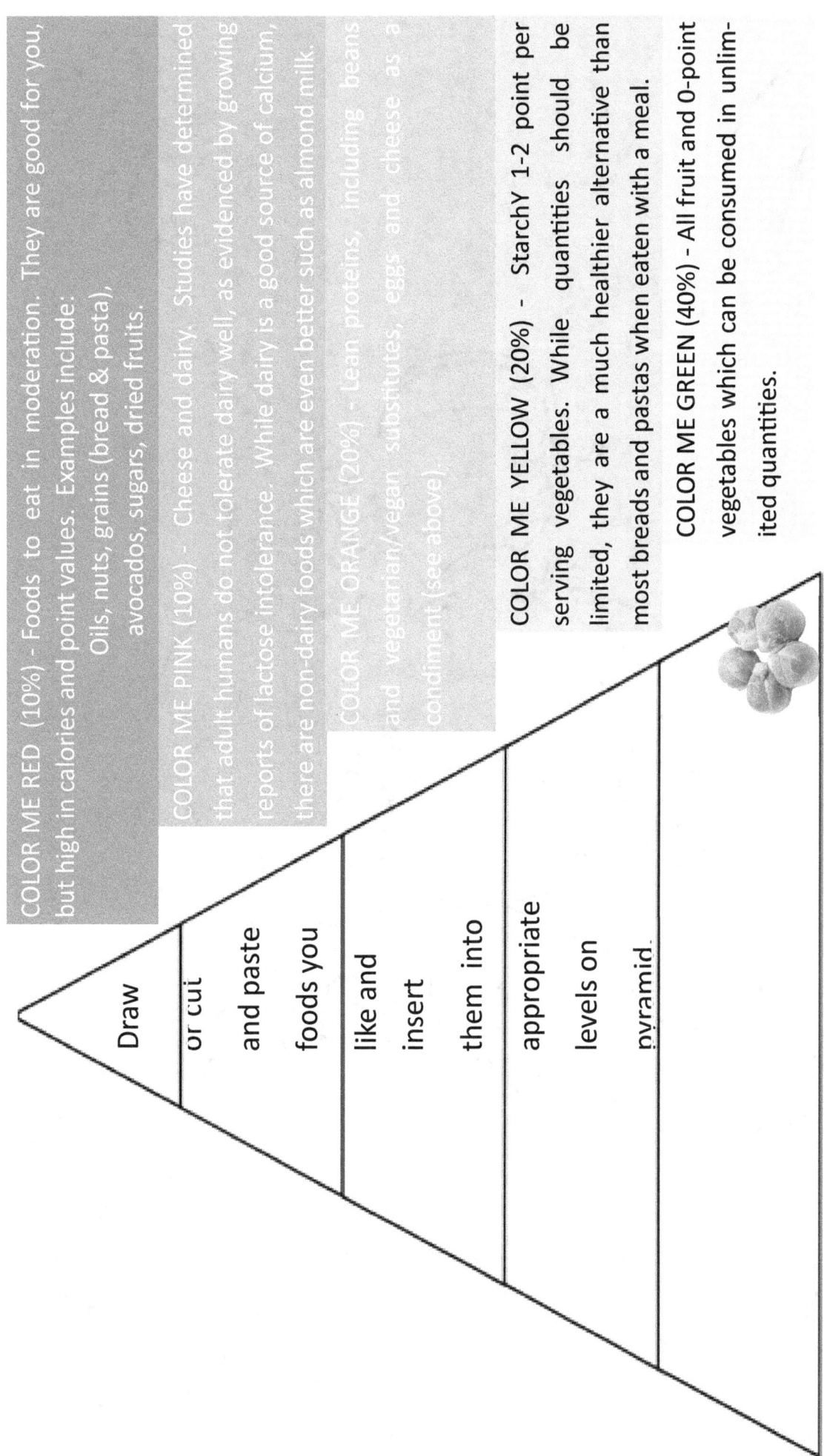

Draw

or cut

and paste

foods you

like and

insert

them into

appropriate

levels on

pyramid.

EXAMPLE: I love brussels sprouts so I copied and pasted a small image of this 0-point vegetable onto the pyramid.

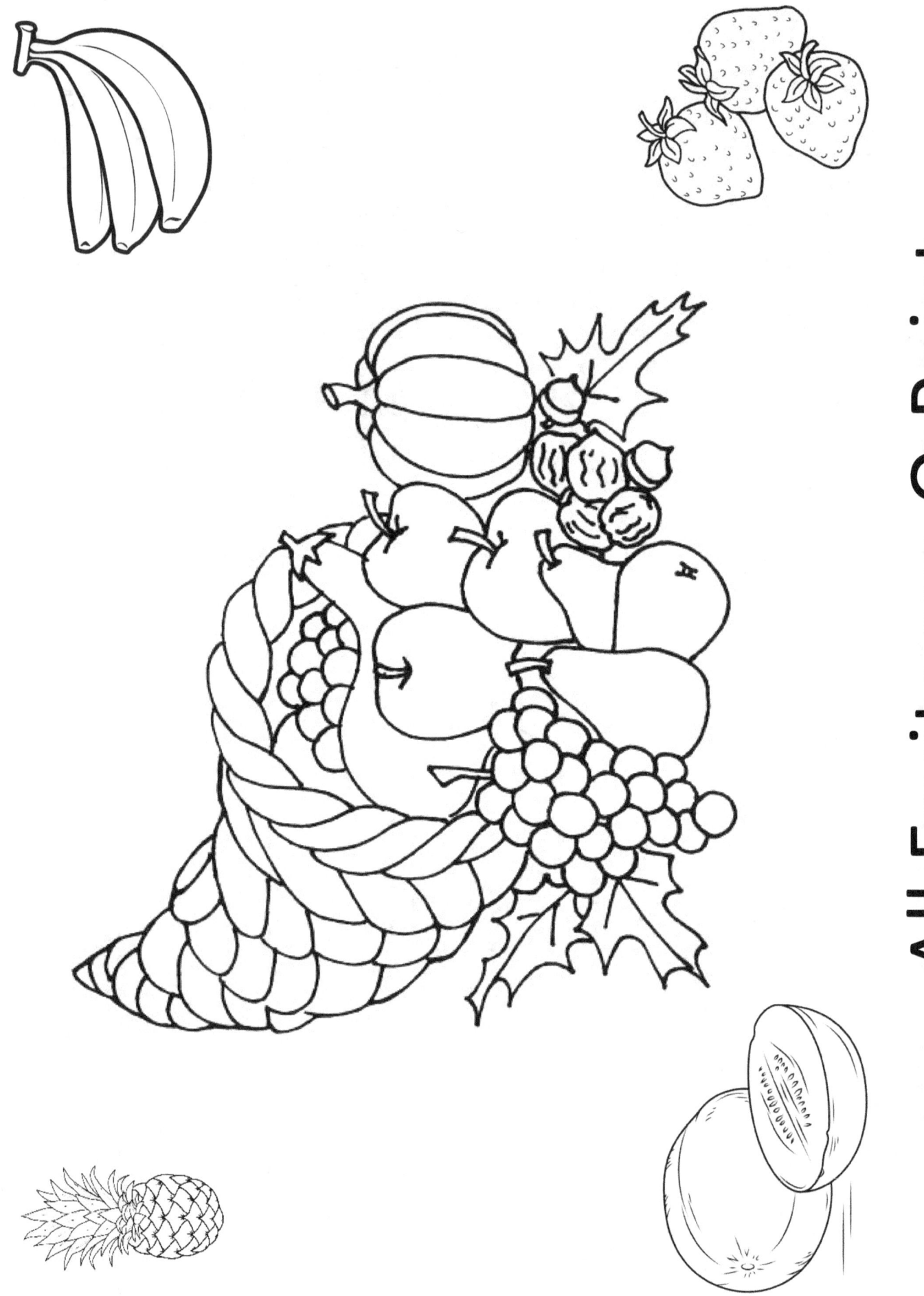

All Fruits are O-Point

-2-

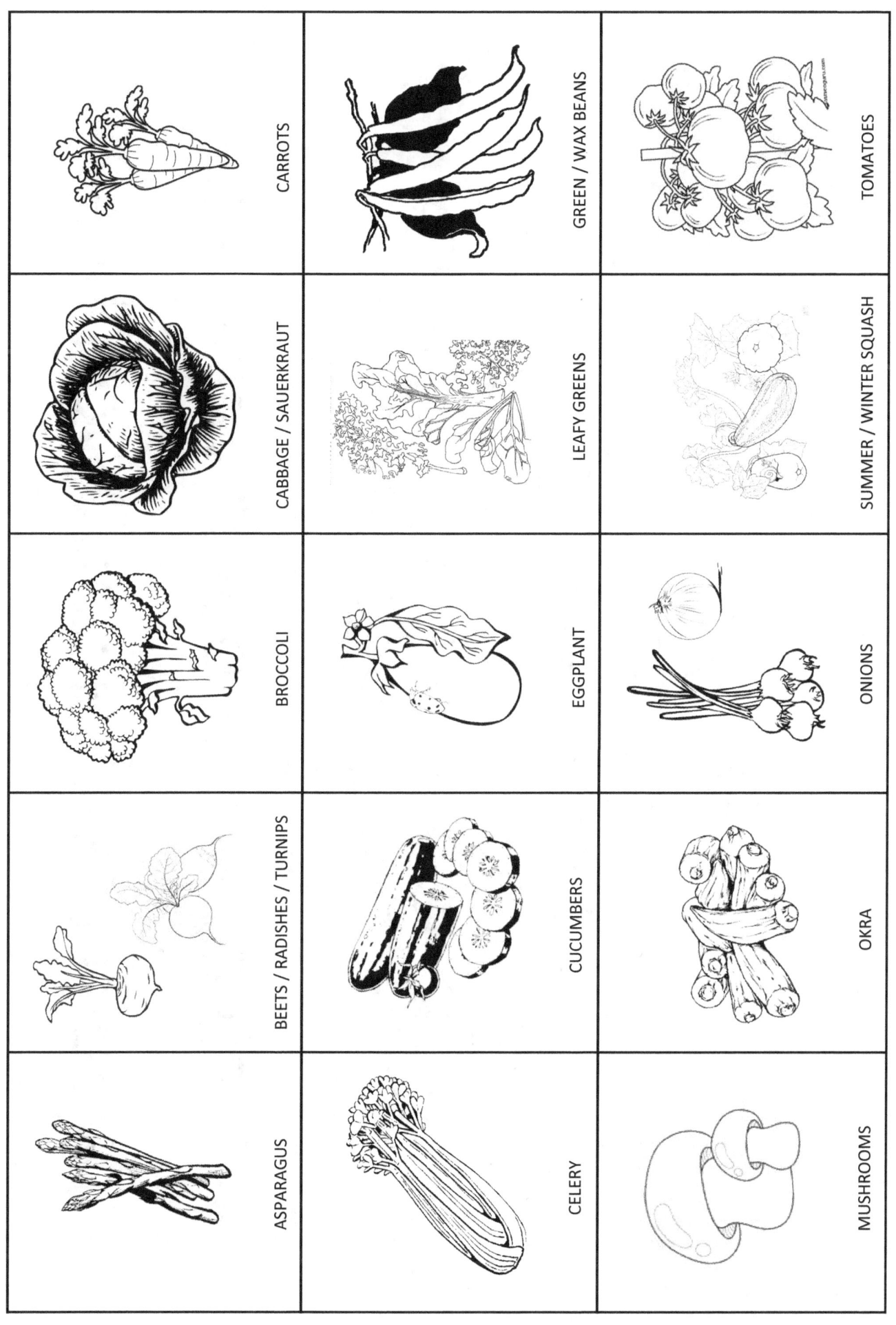

CARROTS

GREEN / WAX BEANS

TOMATOES

CABBAGE / SAUERKRAUT

LEAFY GREENS

SUMMER / WINTER SQUASH

BROCCOLI

EGGPLANT

ONIONS

BEETS / RADISHES / TURNIPS

CUCUMBERS

OKRA

ASPARAGUS

CELERY

MUSHROOMS

# O-Point Vegetables

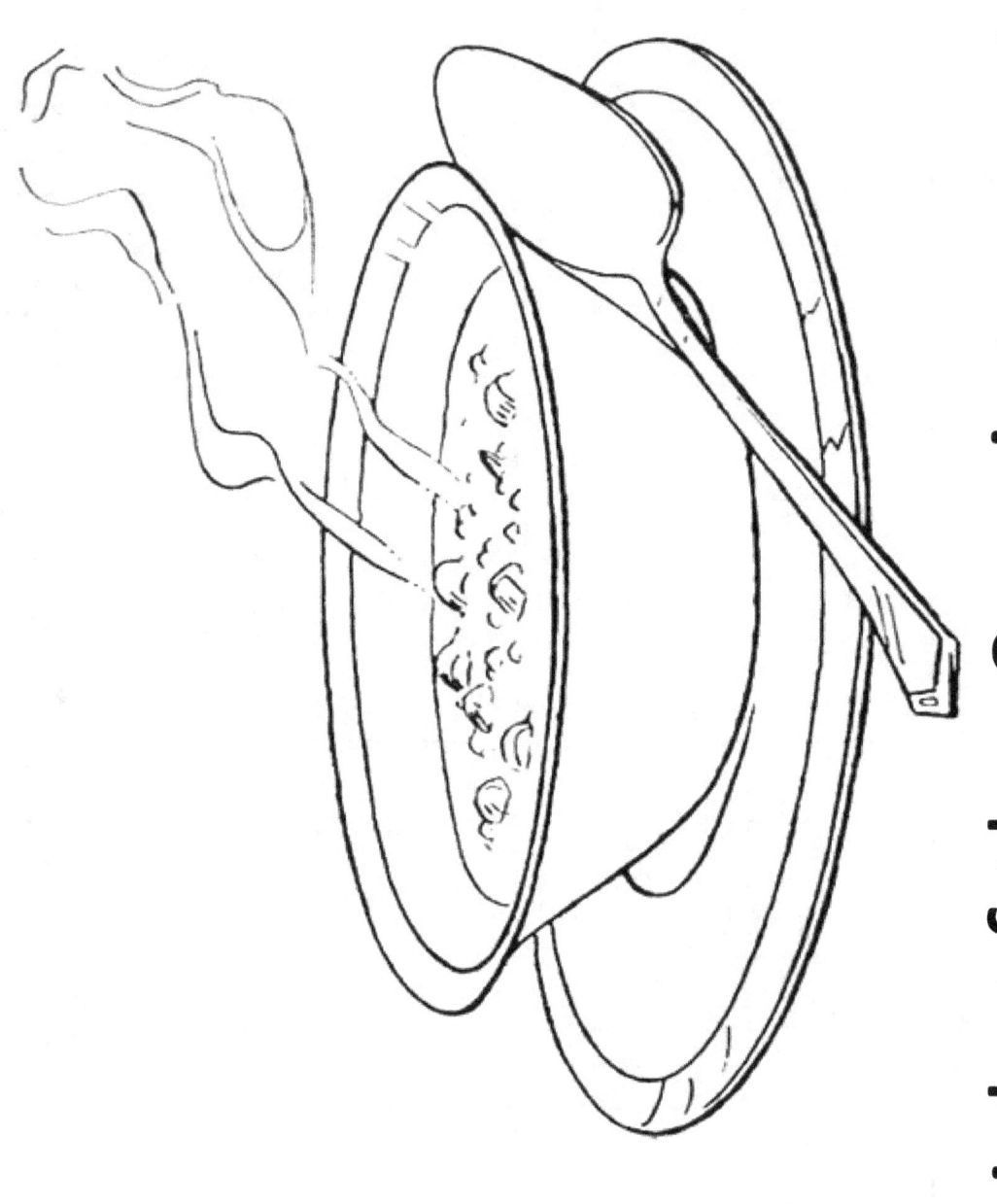

Which of the 0-point vegetables
would make a soup you like?

| | | |
|---|---|---|
| BEANS, DRIED | CORN | |
| | LENTILS | PARSNIPS |
| | | POTATOES, WHITE |
| | PEAS, DRIED | PEAS, FRESH |
| | POTATOES, SWEET | |

# 1-3 Points Per Serving Vegetables

-5-

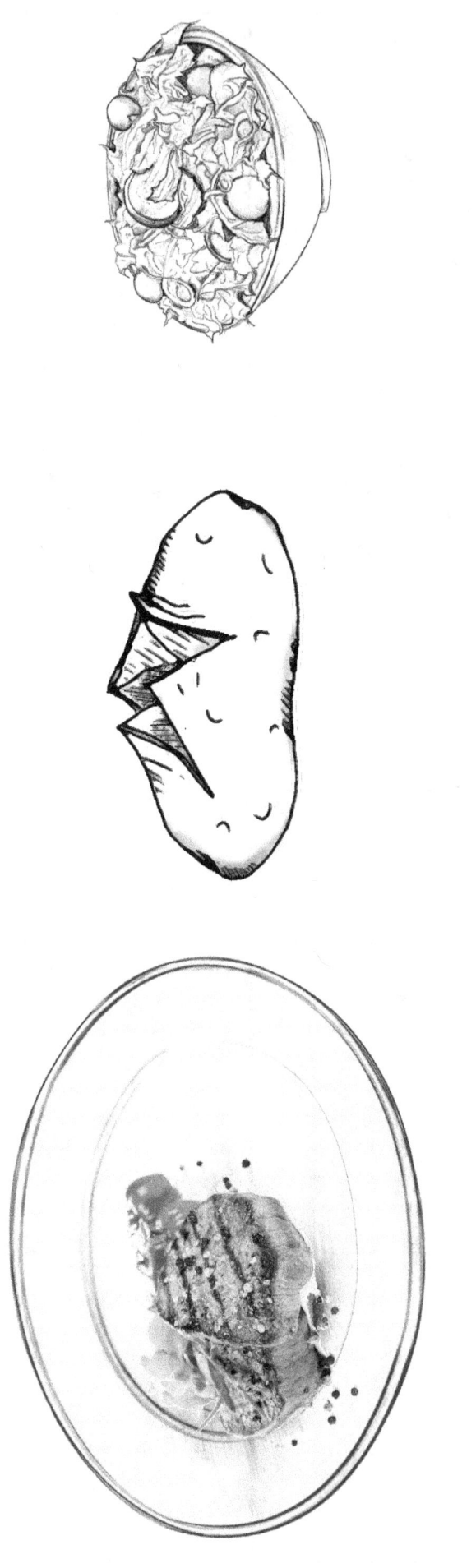

3 oz. lean protein    1/2 C. starch vegetable    0-point salad

A healthy lunch or dinner meal

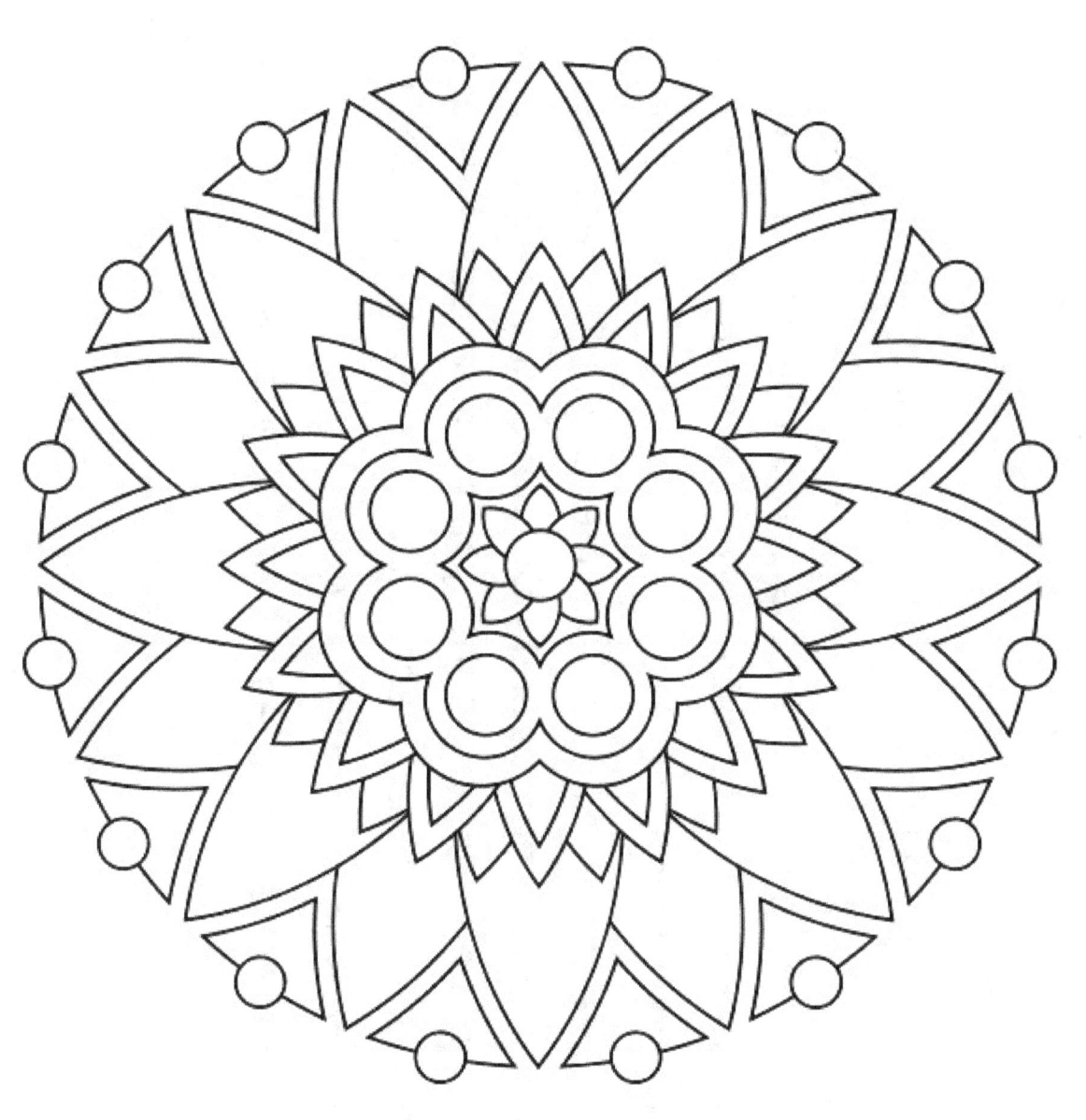

One way to take your mind off being hungry is to color a mandala such as the one above.

# Let Your Fingers

## Do the Walking

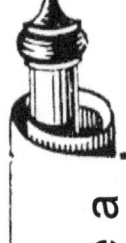

Walking a labyrinth is considered by many to be a spiritual practice. It occurred to me that some of you may not be able at the present time to actually go outdoors and physically walk a labyrinth, or there may not be one near you.

Use a pencil to follow the labyrinth maze below from beginning to end. Do so slowly, meditatively. Repeat an affirmation that you have chosen silently or aloud. Or you may want to listen to the "Shape Shifting Motivational CD" while drawing.

Either way, relax and enjoy the exercise.

# Labyrinth Meditation

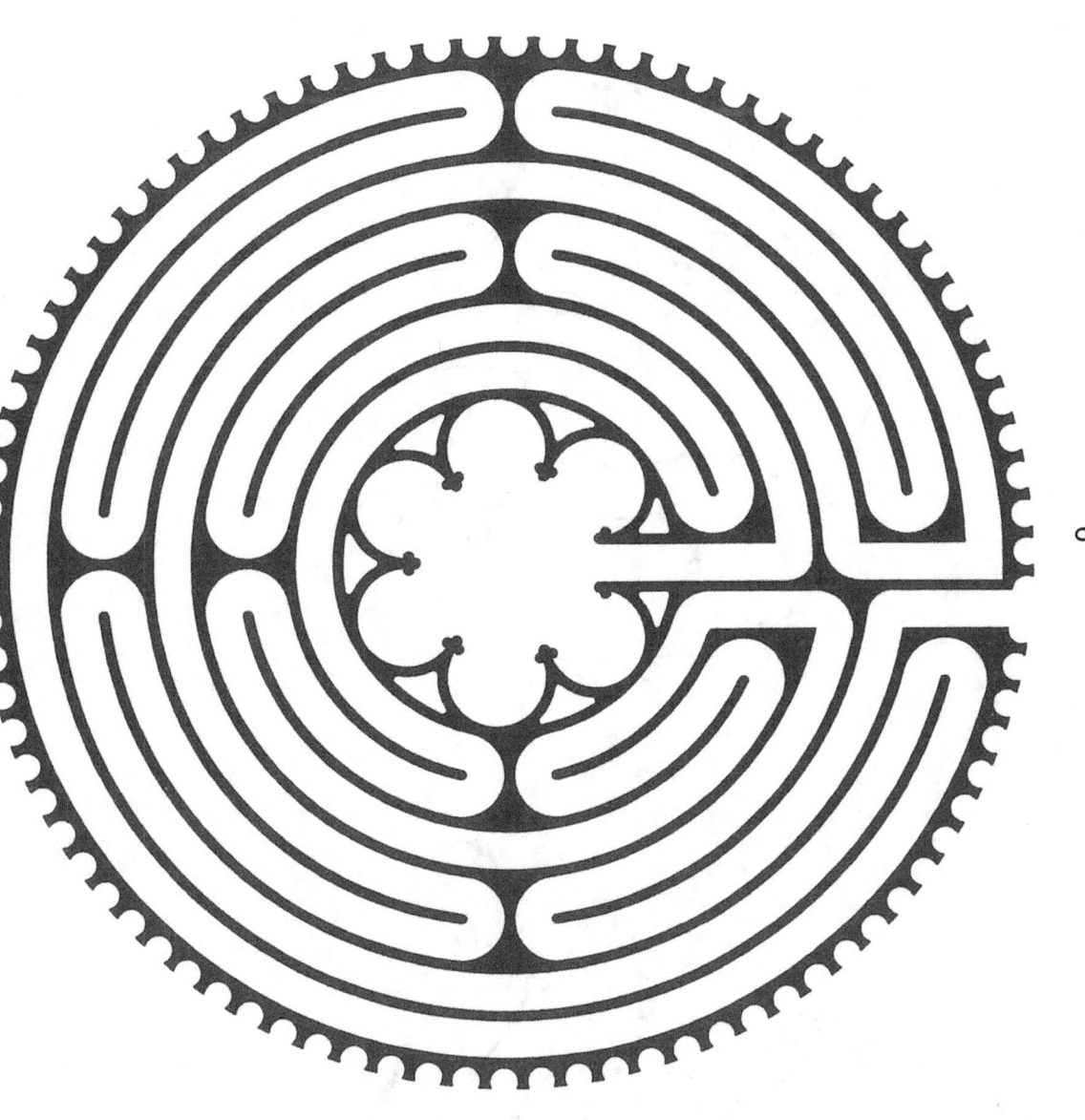

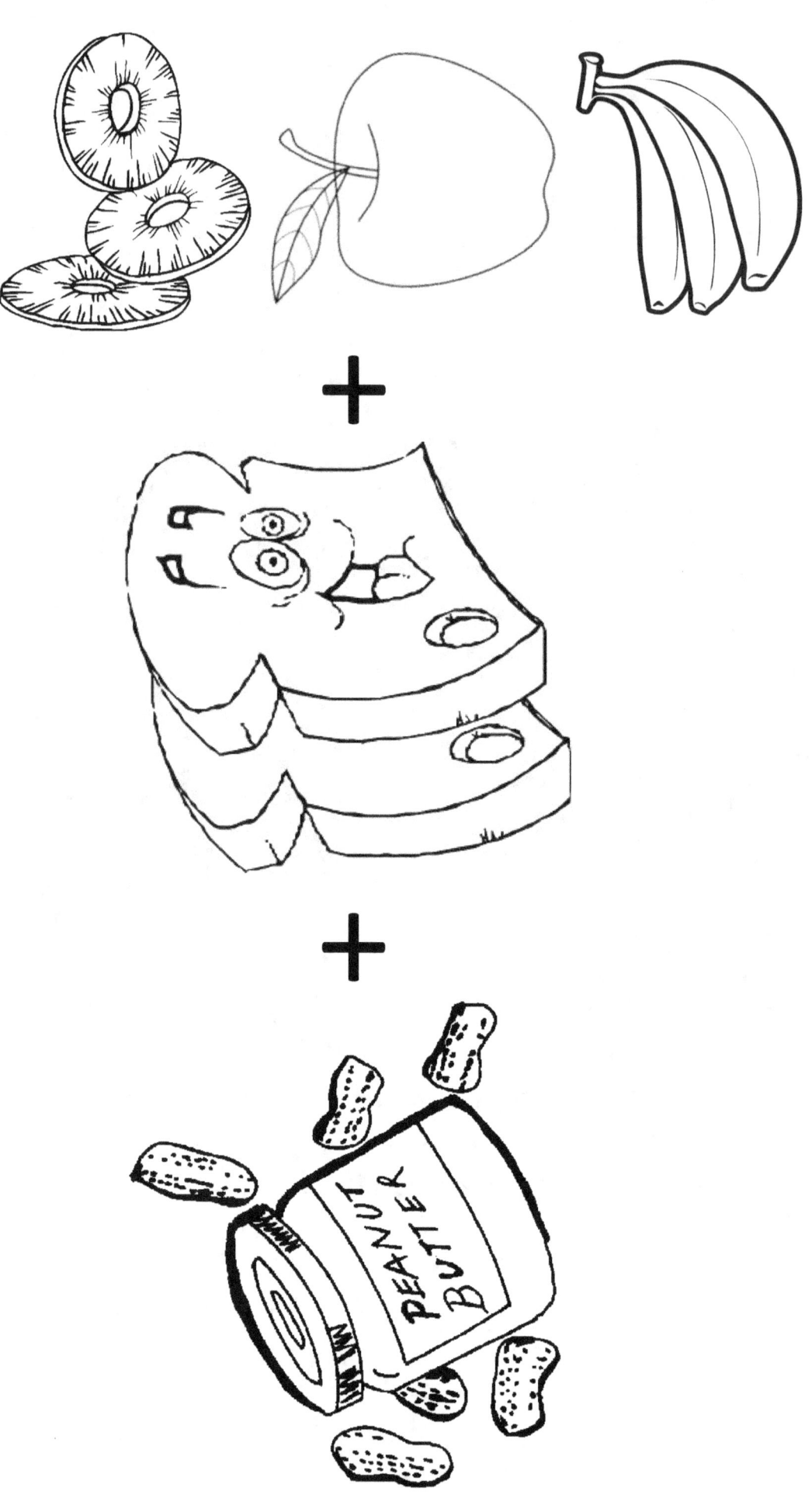

Any Fruit

+

2 sl. High Fiber Bread

A healthy breakfast or snack

1 T. Peanut Butter

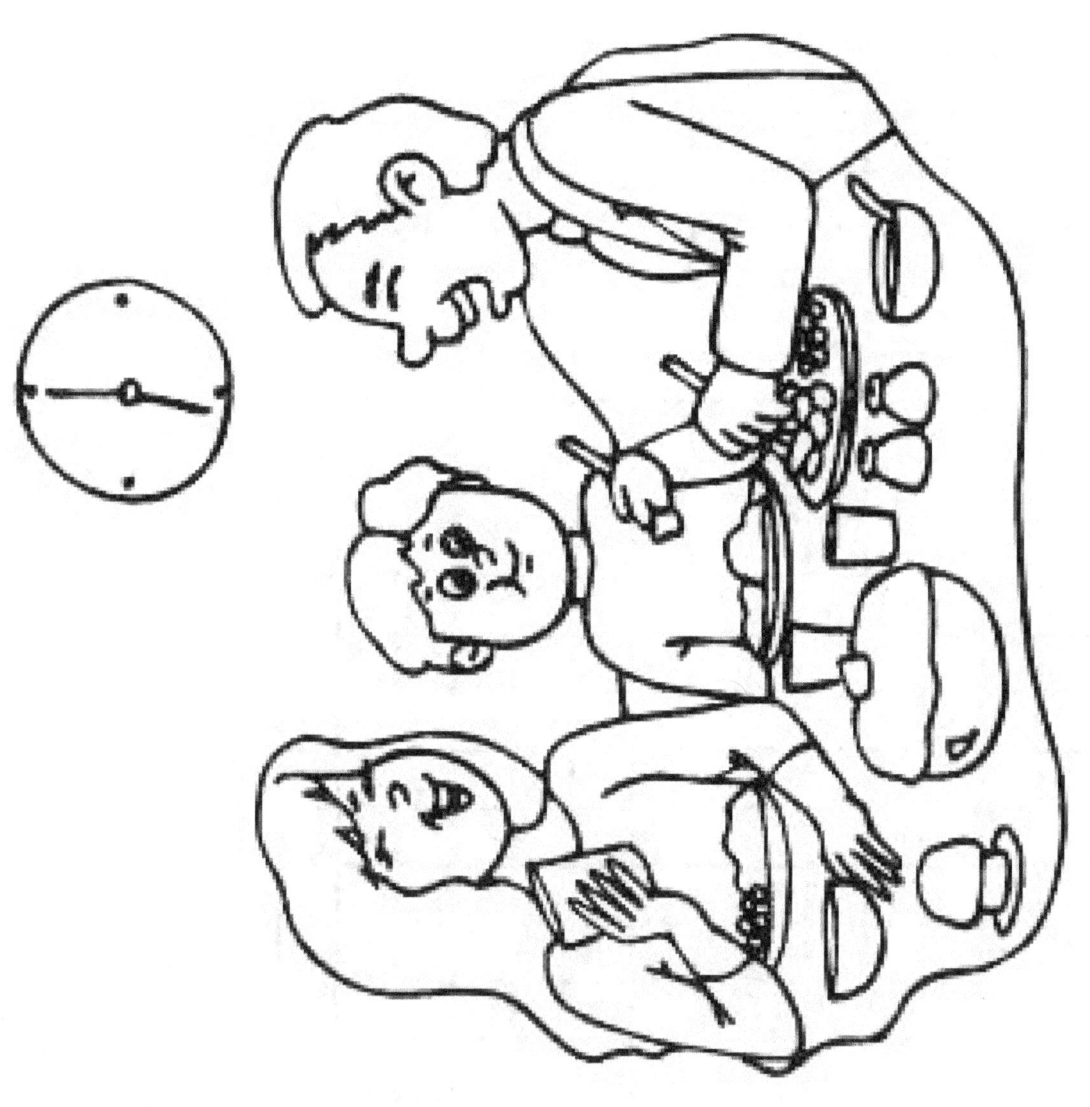

Color this happy family at dinner.

# I AM a Shape Shifter
## Crossword Puzzle

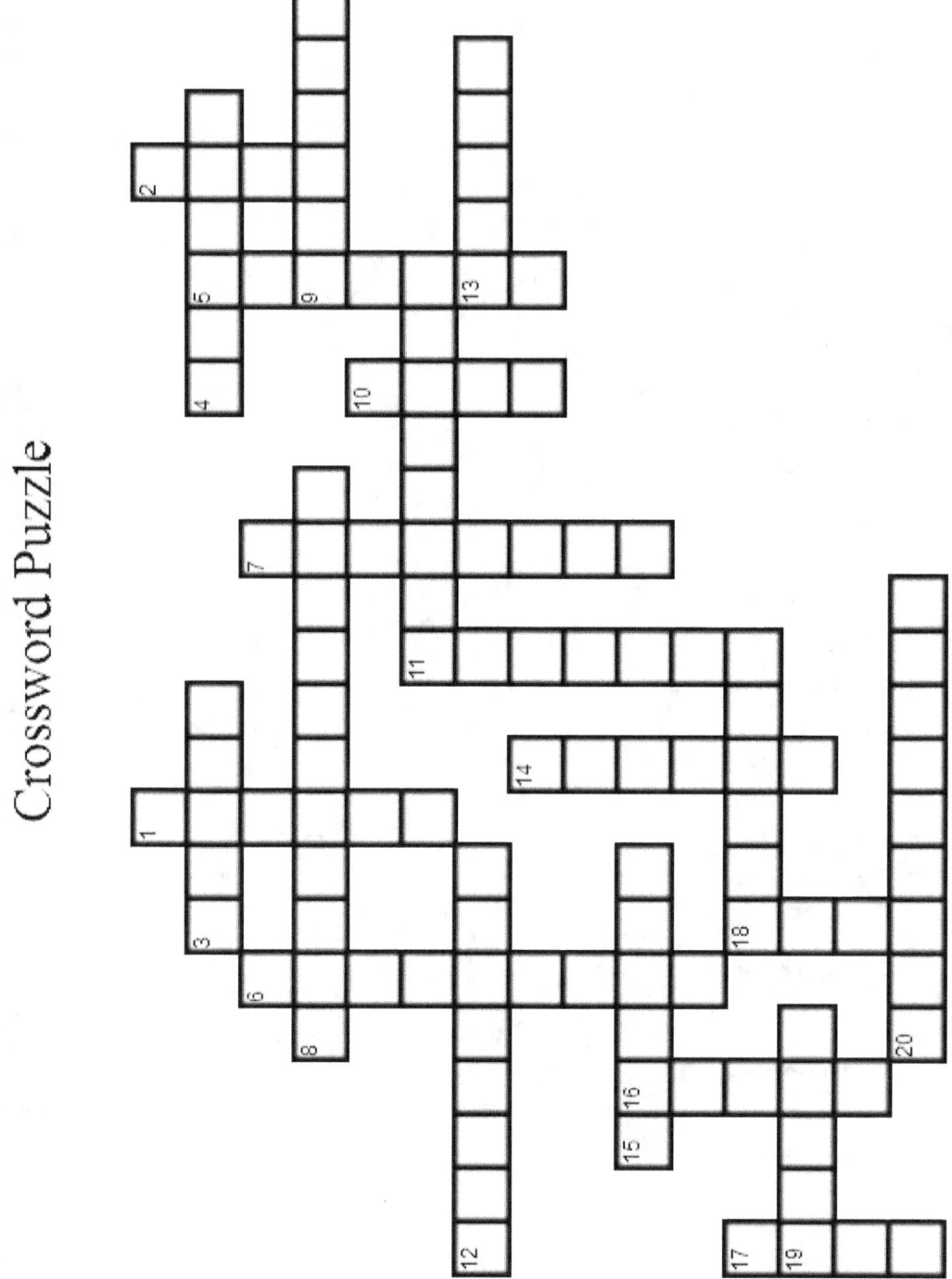

## DOWN

1) Use a diary to analyze your _____ habits.
2) According to "A Course in Miracles", there are only two emotions - fear and _____.
5) Fear can come in many forms, including fear of _____.
6) In addition to physical issues, weight loss involves mental, _____, spiritual and environmental issues.
7) The word "diet" means food and drink regularly _____.
10) One gram of fat has _____ calories.
11) A question to ask when considering a weight loss _____ - "Is it something I can live with long-term?"
14) Weighing and measuring foods are good _____ to develop.
16) Releasing weight is like peeling layers from an _____.
17) Weight is a _____ we put up to protect ourselves.
18) If you _____ it, write it.

## ACROSS

3) Sharon says that she _____ with spices and exotic sauces.
4) It is important to have a clear _____ of what you want to accomplish in any/all areas of your life.
8) _____ is a powerful tool for releasing weight.
9) A "magical" encounter is something we _____ ourselves by our thoughts, words and actions.
11) Stress that affects our actions can be either _____ or negative.
12) The more low point items you eat, the more _____ you can have.
13) Variety is the _____ of life.
15) A baked _____ has more nutrients and less calories than potato chips.
18) When looking at a Food Pyramid you can eat unlimited amounts of foods on the _____ level.
19) Negativity has no power over us unless we _____ it to.
20) Balancing calories or points is like balancing a _____.

Word games were one of the ways my schoolteacher mother taught me how to read and to expand my vocabulary. I still find them to be a fun exercise and hope that you enjoy this puzzle as much as I enjoyed creating it.

Answers are upside down on the bottom of page 19, but please test your memory on what you have read by trying to answer the questions before looking at the answers.

Crossword created using www.puzzle-maker.com/CW/ program.

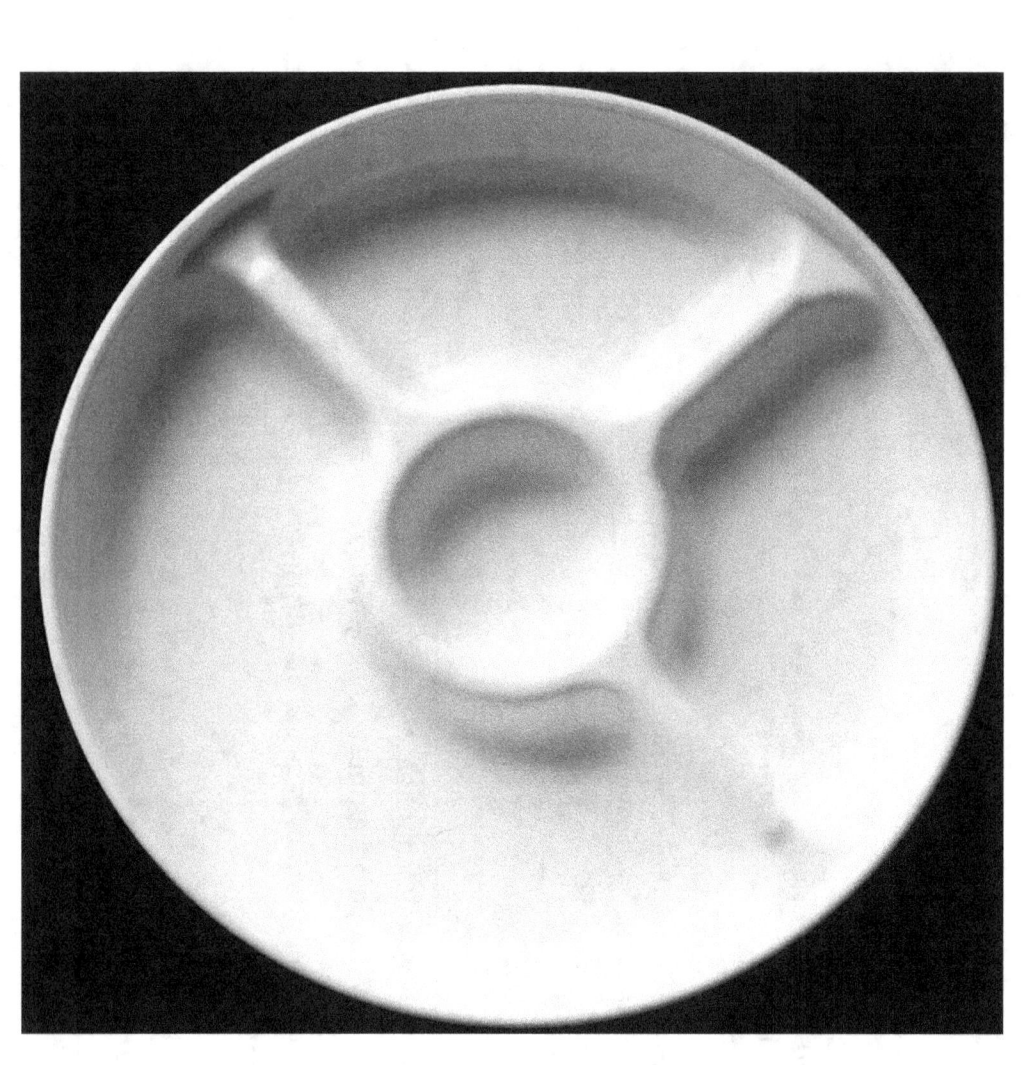

Fill this plate with your favorite vegetable, starch and protein

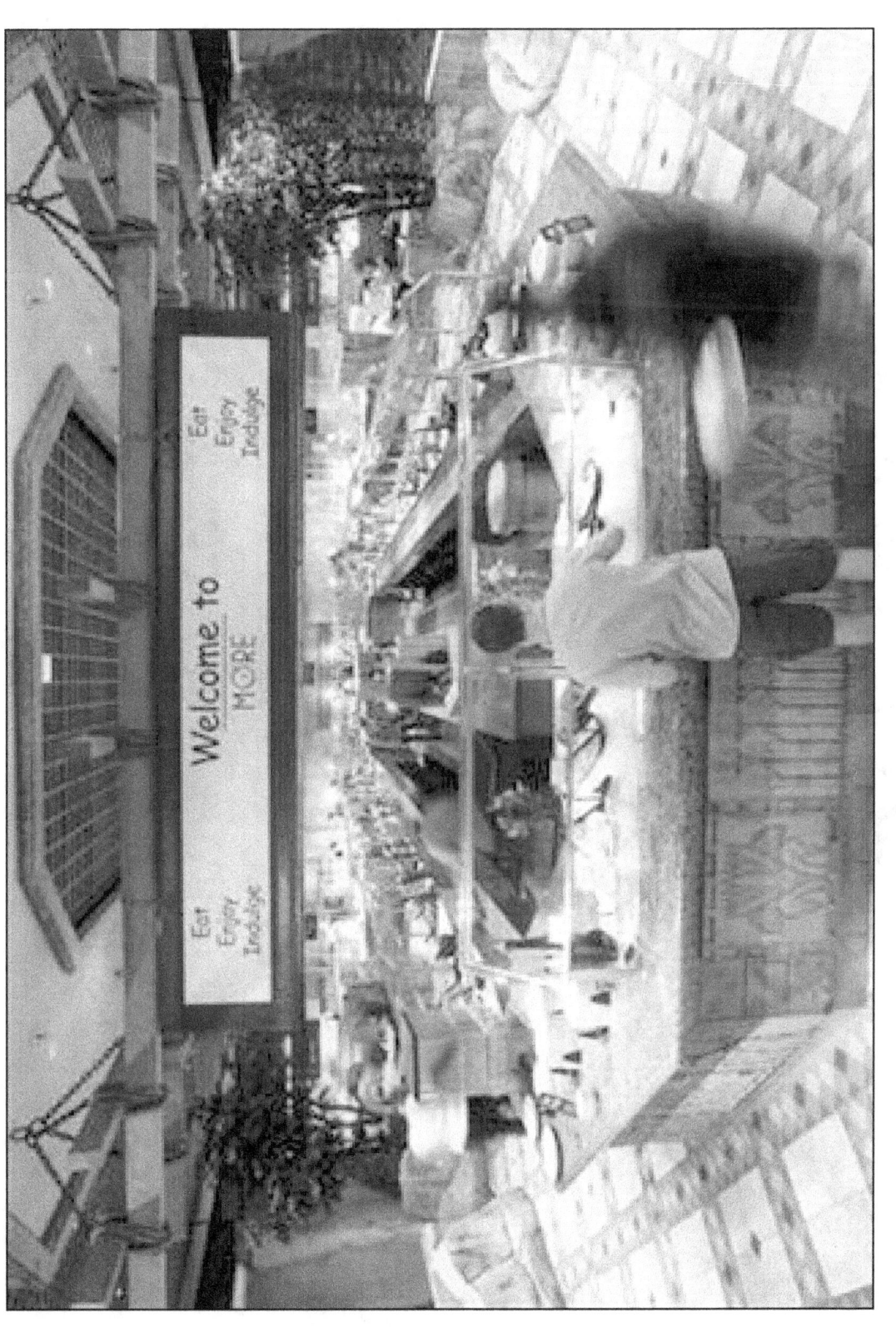

All you can eat buffets can be a disaster to a weight loss program.

Bet you can't choose small amounts of 3-4 items.

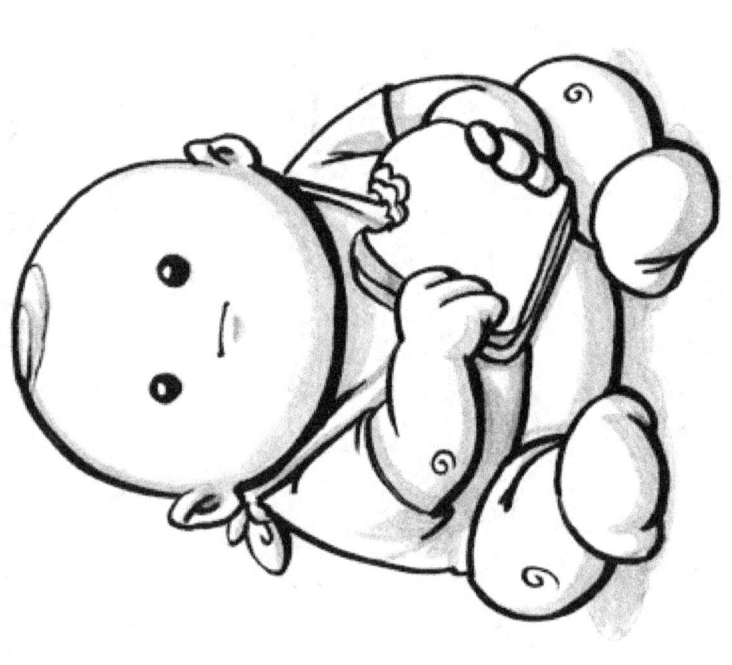

## INTERGENERATIONAL OBESITY

Obesity often runs in families.

Obesity is usually not genetic

Obesity is usually caused by improper diet habits.

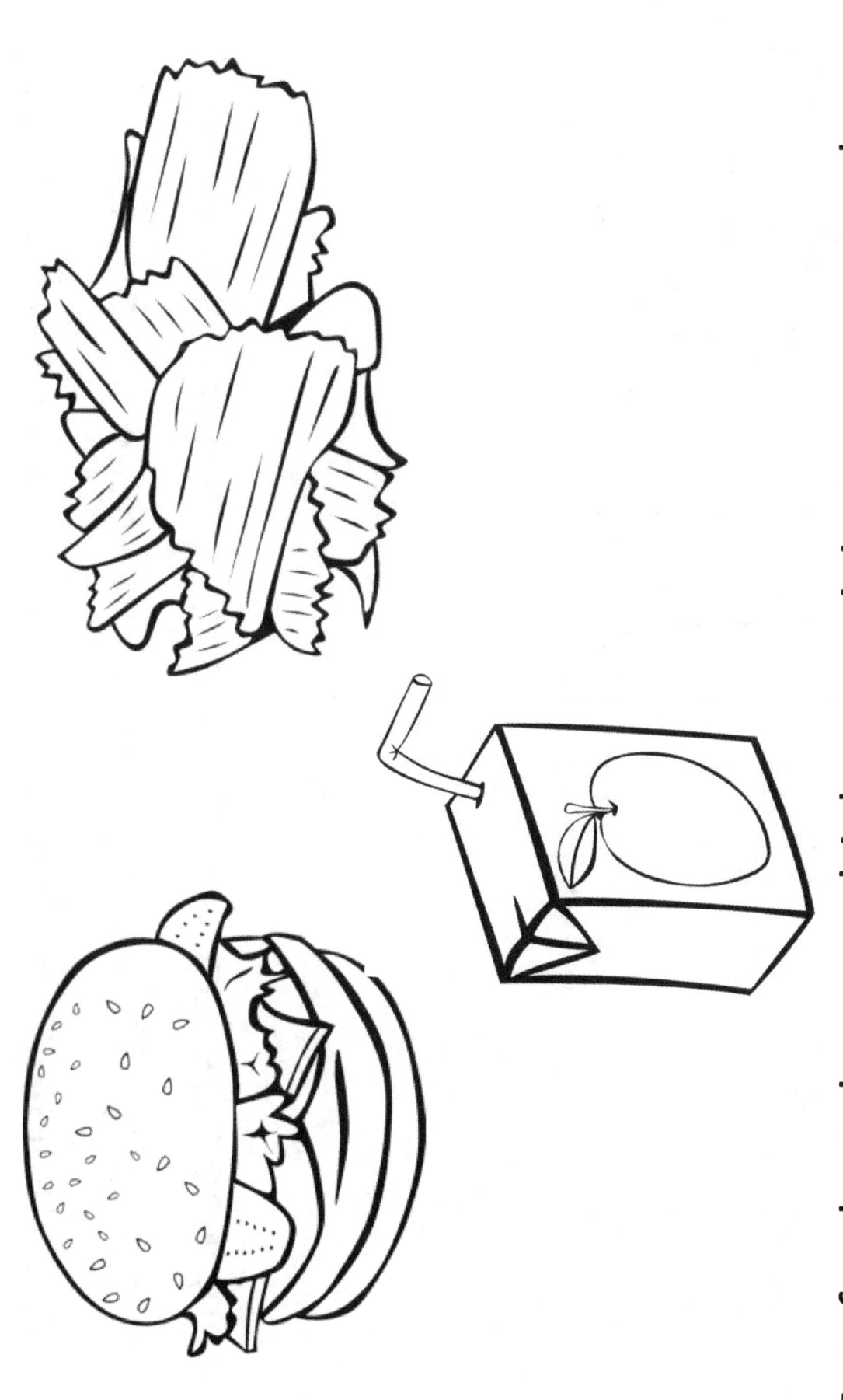

Fast foods and sugary drinks, even juices, are among the worst sources of added calories and fat.

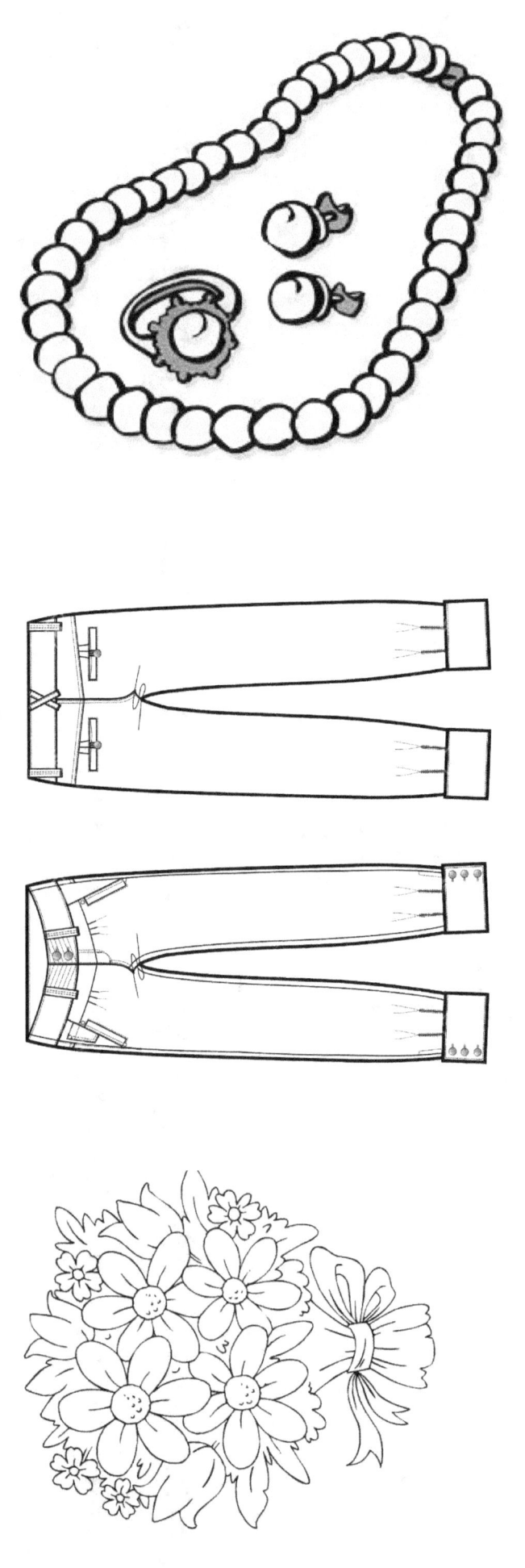

Often, when we lose weight, we reward ourselves with—food!

A good way to change that mindset is by focusing on

something tangible that does not involve food. Some things

that might be appropriate are shown above and below. Put a set amount of money in a jar or piggy bank for each pound you lose.

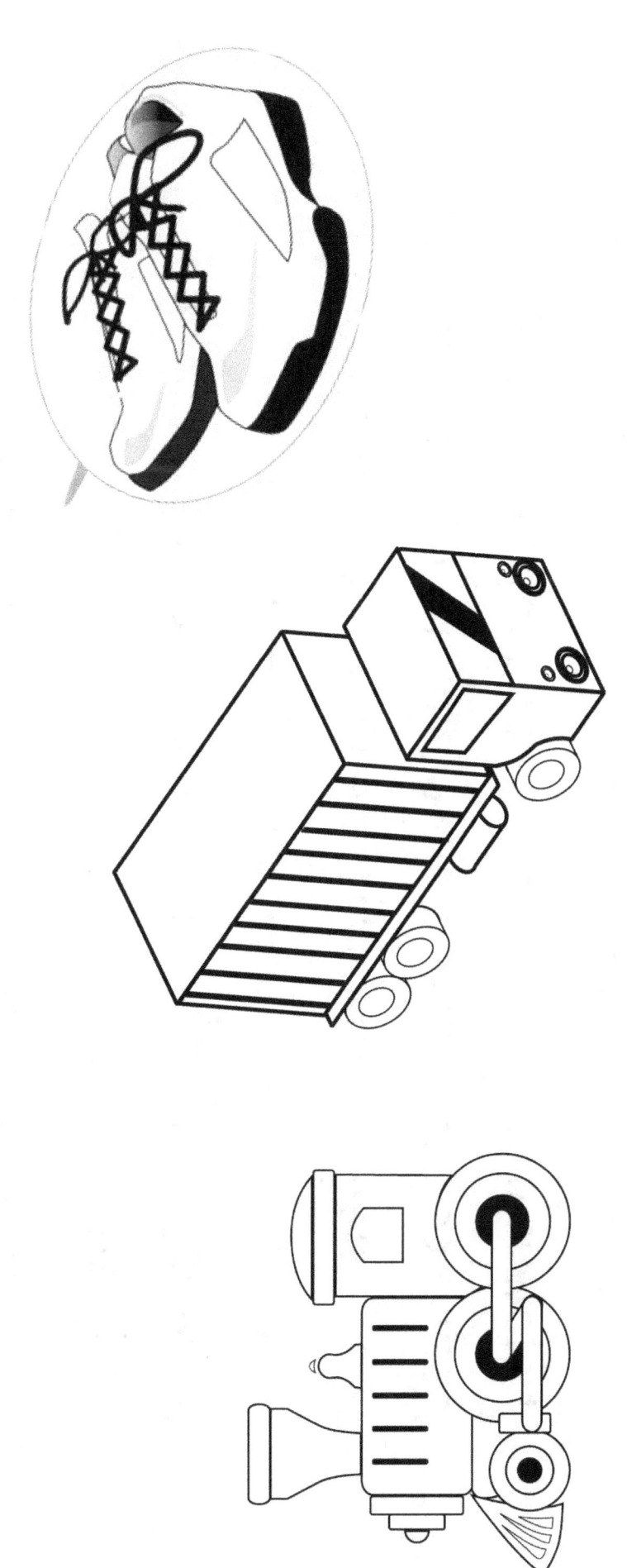

I hope you have enjoyed this book. The drawing below is one that I have used on my Creative Visualization charts. I take a picture of my face, reduce it to a size needed to cover the drawing of the woman's face; then color the rest of the picture. It was an amazingly effective visualization for me and I hope it will benefit you, as well.

Namaskar (the Divinity in me recognizes the Divinity in you).

# What would it take to make you happy?

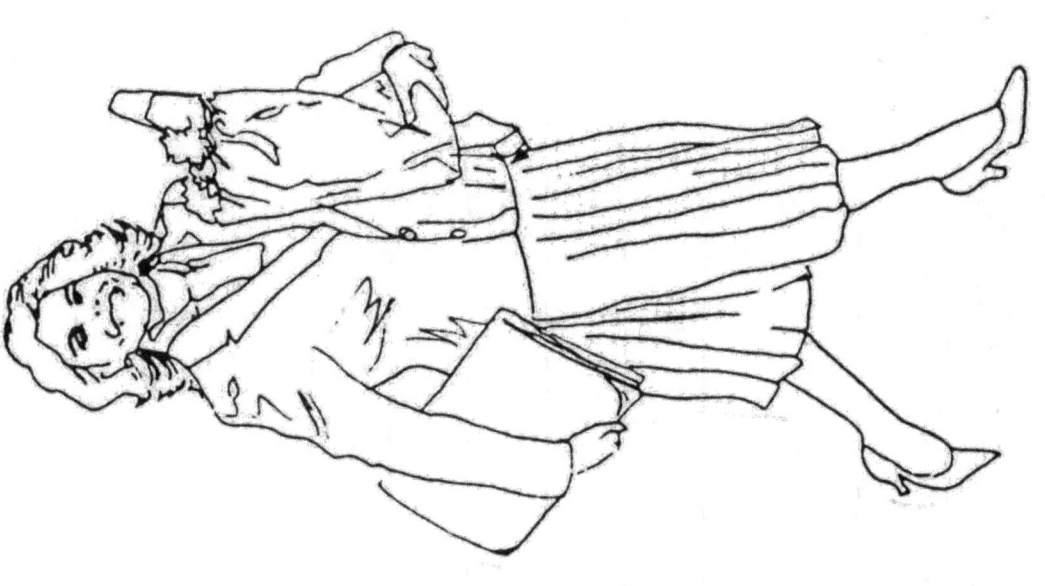

# What foods go on your list?

| 0-Point Vegetables | Starchy Vegetables | Proteins | Dairy | Other |
|---|---|---|---|---|
| | | | | |
| | | | | |
| | | | | |
| | | | | |
| | | | | |
| | | | | |
| | | | | |
| | | | | |

After working with this coloring book I realized that I _____